Fasting: Fast Track to Fat Loss

Fasting: Fast Track to Fat Loss

Josh Bryant and Adam benShea

Table of Contents

Introduction

Fasting is the intentional refrainment from consumption for a time period. Most often, a fast is abstaining from food. After a meal is digested and absorbed, the period until the next meal is eaten is known as a fast. So, it could be overnight, over part of a day, or much longer.

Recently, intermittent fasting has received attention on social media apps, between sets at your local iron pit, and in casual conversations around the pool at neighborhood parties. A lot of discussions on the topic appear to be rich with hyperbole, embellishment, and tales of transcendent journeys through metaphysical forests of personal discovery.

To help you navigate your way through this jungle of data, we offer this project as a compass. Use it to locate the key points and then refer to them often, to avoid getting lost in the overwhelming inundation of online information.

Although it is trending hotter than your favorite reality television star's booze binge down in Old Mexico, fasting is nothing new. It has a rich history in health, spiritual, and political movements.

Long praised as the paragon of wisdom, Greek philosophy is filled with examples of legendary thinkers espousing the benefits of fasting.

Well before he achieved acclaim as one of the greatest thinkers of the ancient world, Plato was a talented grappler who competed in the Isthmian Games. In fact, his name, Platon, means "broad shouldered," in reference to the boulder-like shoulders he developed through hours of wrestling. His balanced life of rigorous physical training and demanding cerebral activity required a rare degree of awareness. To perform at a high level, Plato said, "I fast for greater physical and mental efficiency."

Similarly, the famous Greek historian Plutarch suggested using fasting as a therapeutic treatment.

The father of modern medicine and the namesake of the Hippocratic Oath (requiring a physician to uphold certain ethical standards), Hippocrates prescribed fasting to treat a wide range of ailments from cardiovascular disease to diabetes.

While there are those who suspect or presume that scientific medical claims and religious ideas are categorically opposed to one another, the two fields are in agreement on this topic and emphatic in their call for the benefits associated with fasting.

Religion is overflowing with examples of prophetic figures and disciplined ascetics who practiced, and called for, fasting as a means to purify oneself and draw closer to God.

In Judaism, fasting has been, and continues to be practiced as, part of religious rituals and holidays. There are many fast days in Judaism; the best known is Yom Kippur, or the Day of Atonement. Curiously, fasting on Yom Kippur includes not just abstaining from food, but also refraining from drink, bathing, and sexual relations.

Fasting serves as a means to achieve a form of purification for greater spiritual insight. It also allows the religious believer to draw closer to the prophet, because fasting is a recurrent theme across the prophetic experience.

In the Bible, Moses fasts for 40 days before receiving the commandments from God at Mt. Sinai. Similarly, during his temptation in the desert, Jesus fasted for 40 days.

Early Christian ascetics practiced fasting as a means to draw closer to Jesus. The concept of *imitatio Christi*, or the imitation of Christ, has been an ideal within Christianity since the first century. Many devoted followers of Jesus and his teachings used various forms of renunciation of worldly desires and pursuits as a means to mimic the martyrdom of Jesus. In a manner similar to Jesus turning away from the world by giving up his material body, the believer who emulates Jesus looks beyond the finite realm and toward the infinite by abandoning the trappings of the profane, or secular, realm.

The practice of fasting is one of the more prominent and demonstrable ways of imitating Jesus. The ultimate aim of Christian believers who practice worldly renunciation is to draw closer to Jesus's sacredness and, in the process, be blessed by their sheer proximity to his being. From this perspective, fasting allows one to become more holy.

In Islam, the prophet Muhammad was a strong advocate for fasting, and the central text, the Qur'an, states: "To fast is best for you, if only you knew." From the seventh century to present day, Muslims worldwide fast from sunrise to sunset during the holy month of Ramadan. Many Muslims fast regularly on both Monday and Thursday. Moreover, in the collection of sayings of Muhammad, it is recorded that a believer should fast three times monthly.

Of course, fasting is also prevalent in Buddhism. Siddhartha Gautama's experience with fasting was a crucial part of his journey toward attaining enlightenment and reaching his status as the Buddha ("the Awakened One"). Early on in his spiritual development, Gautama practiced a type of strict fasting that allowed for only one kernel of rice a day. This practice resulted in the Buddha becoming so emaciated that his bones showed through his skin. With time, the Buddha broke from this type of extreme fasting and focused on a more balanced meditative focus. Eventually, the Buddha taught a middle path between sensual overindulgence and severe asceticism.

Therein is an important lesson: Prolonging the act of purposeful food denial may hinder spiritual progress, but the ability to fast for a limited duration was, and remains, an important step on the journey to spiritual awakening.

Still today, monastic followers of Buddhism have their last meal before noon and will then fast until the following morning. In Theravada Buddhism (which is considered to be the oldest existing school of Buddhism), fasting falls under a type of ascetic practice known as *dhutanga*, or "shaking up." Fasting, then, can be thought of as a type of spiritual invigoration, like a metaphysical cold shower, leaving you acute, awake, and aware. Popular with Thai forest monks, the idea is that various forms of fasting provide a means to cultivate deeper spiritual practices and detachment from material goods.

Much like what you see in Buddhism and Christian ascetic practices, fasting in Hinduism represents the denial of physical needs for the purpose of acquiring spiritual gains. According to Hindu scriptures, fasting allows one to become closer to the Absolute through the process of creating a more balanced relationship between body and soul. There is a belief in Hinduism that food consumption equates to the gratification of the senses, while fasting elevates the senses to a place of contemplation.

Depending on their adherence to a particular deity inside of the broad spectrum of worship that falls under the umbrella term of Hinduism, adherents may fast at different times during the week or month and during a wide array of festivals (with the nine-day holiday of Navaratri being one of the more popular examples).

A popular, and very ancient, Indian medical system known as Ayurveda is seen by some as related to the cultural tradition of Hinduism. The Ayurvedic view of health is based on the belief that many diseases are caused by the buildup of toxic materials in the digestive system. To keep a person healthy, it is necessary to have a regular cleansing of toxic materials. Fasting gives the digestive organs a rest, and the body, as a whole, is cleansed, and maybe even corrected. During this Ayurvedic fast for health, lemon juice is allowed as a means to keep things flowing.

Taking the concept of fasting a step further, Ayurvedic thought asserts that at various times changes in the fluid contents of the body may create emotional imbalances. From this perspective, fasting can be used as a means to treat emotional stress and irritability.

Fasting has also been used as a tool for pushing societal change. Famously, in the 20th century, the well-known activist Mahatma Gandhi (who was born to a Hindu family) used fasting in the form of a hunger strike to effect political change. Interestingly, the performance of *not* doing something (in this case, eating) has been shown to be successful in making real change.

From a more general humanitarian perspective, the pangs of hunger experienced during fasting can create greater empathy. Those who are more privileged can acquire a better understanding of those who may not have enough to eat. From this experience of empathy, there may be room for compassion, and when there is compassion, you are more likely to use your strength to be a source of strength for others.

The sheer prevalence of fasting across religious examples raises the question of why this practice is in place. There are three possible theories about its purpose: one, a spiritual cleansing, two, a means to have a transcendent experience, or, three, a method of producing a new vitality.

Whether your religious ritual is regular attendance at a neighborhood church, your preferred spiritual awakening is hallucinogens in an Amazonian rainforest, or your means of meditative practice is 30 minutes on the heavy bag in your garage followed by a six-pack of Shiner Bock, the desire to have a cleansing, uplifting, and invigorating practice remains consistent.

Fasting provides all of that while also offering demonstrable physical improvement.

There is actually a long history of the use of fasting as a tool for increased athletic performance. Back in ancient Greece, athletes utilized fasting to prepare their bodies for the rigors of the Olympic Games. The mathematician and philosopher Pythagoras fasted for 40 days ahead of his exams at the Alexandria School. After this he prescribed fasting to his pupils because of the noticeable increased mental clarity and physical strength.

In more recent times, the great football player, sprinter, martial artist, and Olympic bobsledder Herschel Walker has practiced a form of intermittent fasting for decades. He skips breakfast and lunch, eating only a simple meal at dinner. Moreover, when Walker was preparing for his MMA debut (at almost 50 years old), there would be instances when he would complete seven hours of grappling and kickboxing training while not eating for three or four days.

Herschel Walker is by no means the only elite athlete who makes use of intermittent fasting. The former UFC welterweight and middleweight champion Georges St-Pierre had a bout of ulcerative colitis (a bowel disease which leads to inflammation in the digestive tract) that caused him to rethink his nutrition plan and ultimately resulted in his practice of fasting. Although there are certain foods that upset his stomach, St-Pierre is able to eat them so long as he keeps his food consumption inside of an eight-hour window. This allows him to continue eating ice cream, for instance.

In addition, three times a year St-Pierre will fast for five days con-secutively, during which time he will drink only water. This allows his body to get into a state of autophagy (described below), where his body burns bad cells. It should be noted that during these lengthy fasts St-Pierre continues to train, sometimes even twice a day.

Outside of the Octagon and inside of Tinseltown, actor, lifter, and former pro football player Terry Crews has become a vocal advocate for intermittent fasting. Introduced to the practice by UFC legend Randy Couture, Crews follows the 16:8 method (described below), where he eats in an eight-hour window between 2:00 and 10:00 p.m. Crews, who is known for his comedic timing and lean muscular build, has undoubtedly found that intermittent fasting is serving his physical prowess and mental sharpness.

Cleary, fasting can be beneficial to your spiritual being, but it can also clear your mind and strengthen your physical body.

So, let's talk about the ways in which you can use intermittent fast-ing to lean out for that long weekend on Florida's panhandle, harden up for the local toughman contest, and just look better naked.

Chapter 1:What is Intermittent Fasting?

On an intermittent fasting eating style, you cycle between periods of fasting and eating. For example, you might fast for 16 hours per day, which means you don't eat during that time. And you then consume all your calories in an eight-hour feeding window.

Thus, intermittent fasting doesn't dictate *which* foods you should consume or how much of them (like most diets do). Instead, it's about *when* you consume those foods.

There are various forms of intermittent fasting. We'll cover the method that we recommend in more detail throughout the upcoming sections, but to give you a brief overview, here are three popular styles that have the results to back them up:

- LeanGains by Martin Berkhan, a method during which you fast for 14 to 16 hours per day and eat your foods in a 10- to 8-hour feeding window.
- Eat-Stop-Eat by Brad Pilon, a method in which you fast for 24 hours once or twice per week and follow your regular nutrition plan for the rest of the time.
- The 5:2 diet, an eating style based on eating like you normally would for five days per week and restricting your energy intake to 500 to 600 calories on the other two days.

With most intermittent fasting methods, you abstain from all caloric foods during your "fasting window." But you can—and should—consume non-caloric beverages like water, green tea, and black coffee. However, we recommend avoiding diet soda and any other calorie-free drinks with artificial sweeteners. Keep in mind that dehydration has many adverse effects on your physiology. (More on hydration later.)

Chapter 2: Why Intermittent Fasting Can Help You Get and Stay Lean

Bodybuilders and other physique athletes have long walked around with Tupperware containers wherever they go to get in a meal every few hours. This was based on the antiquated notion that frequent meals would keep their metabolism roaring and simultaneously boost their muscle growth and retention.

The current scientific literature, however, shows that doing so isn't necessary and may even hurt your results. For instance, studies show that intermittent fasting:

- Boosts metabolism by 3.6% to 14%.[1-2] As a result, it'll be easier to get and stay in a calorie deficit, which means your body will burn more body fat for fuel.
- Skyrockets levels of human growth hormone (HGH). Your level of this hormone may increase by as much as five-fold while you're fasting.[3] That's excellent because HGH has powerful fat-burning benefits, and it helps you maintain muscle as you lean down while avoiding the potentially harmful synthetic version of HGH.
- Lowers insulin levels.[4] This makes your body more effective at releasing fat from your fat cells, which means it helps you burn fat. Plus, as an extra benefit, a reduction in insulin levels also impairs the storing of fat.[5-6]
- Increases norepinephrine (noradrenaline) levels.[7] This helps you lose more fat because norepinephrine helps your body use body fat for fuel.

- Decreases hunger. One of the main reasons most diets fail is that they leave you feeling hungry. By eating your foods in a smaller feeding window, you'll experience fewer cravings, making it easier to adhere to your diet.
- Reduces total calorie intake. Researchers have shown that skipping breakfast, which is a form of intermittent fasting, reduces daily calorie intake by up to 400 calories.[8-10] Energy wise, that represents up to 0.8 pound of pure body fat each week![11]

The no-frills truth is that intermittent fasting puts you into a fat-burning state, and you feel less hungry in the process.

So, by following the plan we lay out, you will look better in your three-piece suit for business encounters and more aesthetically pleasing in your birthday suit for intimate ones!

You will also reach your fat loss goals easier and faster with intermittent fasting.

Now, you may have heard from some self-anointed fitness "gurus" that intermittent fasting, or going for extended periods without food, causes muscle wasting. And there are athletes who believe that they'll burn away their muscle mass if they don't consume food every few hours.

Well, what does science say?

The pseudo-scientific skeptics point to an eight-week study published in the *European Journal of Sport Science*.[12] In the study, researchers looked at how intermittent fasting combined with resistance training influenced muscle growth in young, recreationally active men.

All the men followed the same resistance training routine. The only difference was that half of them practiced intermittent fasting, while the other half didn't.

The result?

The regular diet group gained, on average, 2.3 kilograms of lean body mass. In addition, the regular group gained 0.8 kilos of body fat while the fasting group lost 0.6 kilos of body fat. But those who practiced intermittent fasting didn't gain or lose a statistically significant amount of muscle. In other words, those who ate "normally" gained muscle while the intermittent fasting group maintained their muscle mass without gaining additional hypertrophy.

Fundamentalists base their religious interpretation of the Bible on one verse. Similarly, social media diet gurus base their nutritional "philosophy" on one study.

However, whether you're reading a sacred text or a scientific one, context is crucial.

Interestingly, in this study, context is everything. The reason it *appeared* that intermittent fasting is a hindrance to muscle growth is because the fasters consumed around 650 fewer calories per day. Intermittent fasting reduces hunger, causing one to automatically consume fewer calories. That explains why the regular group gained body fat while the fasting group lost body fat.

So, clearly, the fact that those following an intermittent fast gained less muscle was not a result of their intermittent fasting regimen. Rather, it was because they consumed fewer calories, which also caused them to lose fat while the regular group gained some fat.

This once again confirms the fact that every scientist, nutritionist, and "bro scientist" agrees on: If you want to optimize muscle growth, you must be in a caloric surplus. We'll show you exactly how to figure out your ideal calorie intake, based on your situation, goals, and needs!

Now, the second intermittent fasting study provides more insight. In the study, researchers looked at how Ramadan influenced the muscle mass of bodybuilders.[13] As referenced above, Ramadan is the ninth month of the Muslim year, during which strict fasting is observed from sunrise to sunset.

The study showed that when men maintained their regular calorie intake during Ramadan, they would see no adverse changes in muscle mass during the month of daytime fasting. In other words, based on that data, fasting has no or at most minimal negative effects on muscle growth.

As an aside from the numerous scientific studies supporting the benefits of fasting, the well-known Dagestani MMA fighter Khabib Nurmagomedov is a practicing Muslim who fasts during the month of

Ramadan. However, even during the fast, he continues a strict regimen of hard training. Given his impressive performances inside of the cage, it would be difficult to claim that fasting hinders or negatively impacts his athleticism. In fact, you can make the argument that it is one of many tools in his unique training arsenal.

So, returning to science, what can we conclude based on the current scientific literature?

First, calorie intake remains important whether you practice intermittent fasting or not. If you want to gain muscle, you'll have to be in a calorie surplus. And if you want to lose fat, you'll have to be in a calorie deficit.

Second, the data also shows that intermittent fasting causes most people to consume fewer calories automatically. That's why it can be an excellent eating style for those who want to get leaner but have a hard time controlling their food intake.

Since intermittent fasting also pairs with lower insulin levels, an increased metabolism, reduced hunger, and higher norepinephrine levels, it's likely that you will lose more fat on an intermittent fasting eating style than if you would eat "normally," especially if you also optimize your calorie and macro intakes (which we'll show you how to do in an upcoming section).

Now, you can also use intermittent fasting to build muscle. However, it's especially important that you keep track of your calorie intake. This is because the hunger-reducing effects of fasting may cause you to take in too few calories, which would impair muscle growth.

That is, however, not inherently a downside. For example, if you have a hard time controlling your calorie intake while gaining weight or you want to do a lean bulk, intermittent fasting may help you ensure that you don't get too many calories. As a result, you'll be less likely to overeat, which means you may gain less fat while building muscle.

Chapter 3: The Health Benefits of Intermittent Fasting

By now, you have a sense that intermittent fasting will help you look better naked. But, is this at the expense of your health? After all, the "muscle media" often claims that eating small meals every few hours is "best."

In reality, intermittent fasting is not bad for your health. Actually, it can make you healthier. Until recently, people didn't always have access to food. Our ancestors had to deal with periods of food abundance and food shortage. As a result, we've developed metabolic pathways that allow us to function well even for prolonged periods without food.

Better yet, because such cycles were common throughout history, intermittent fasting is a more natural eating style than consuming small meals every few hours. And studies indicate that intermittent fasting is both safe and beneficial.[14] Research shows the following intermittent fasting benefits:

- Reduces inflammation and oxidative stress in your body.[15-16] This likely reduces your risk of all sorts of chronic diseases, such as heart disease and cancer.
- Anti-aging benefits. Research shows that rats who followed an alternate-day fasting eating style lived, on average, 83 percent longer than those who had continuous access to food. [17] What's more, Walter Breuning, who was the world's oldest man when he died at age 114, fasted for 16 hours every day. He attributed his longevity largely to eating in such a way.

- Stimulates autophagy, which is the body's way of cleaning out damaged cells to regenerate newer and healthier ones. This is one reason fasting may improve longevity and health markers.[18]
- Benefits brain health. Shortening your feeding windows stimulates the growth of new nerve cells and the production of BDNF, a key hormone for brain health.[18-19]
- Improves cardiovascular health. Restricting your food intake during most hours of the day may reduce blood triglycerides, body fat percentage, and levels of "bad" LDL cholesterol—all of which reduce your risk of heart disease.[20-21]
- May help reverse the progression of type 2 diabetes, as found in both animal and human studies. This may occur because fasting can lower insulin levels, reduce inflammation, and help burn body fat.[22-23]
- Stem cell regeneration. In a study published in the *Stem Cells* journal, researchers discovered periods of fasting can stimulate stem cell self-renewal, or encourage stem cells to regenerate. Even more exciting is the detail that subjects experienced a 93.7% rise in stem cells after ending their fast.
- Belly fat reduction. Spot reduction is usually passed off as a myth by self-appointed nutritional messiahs; however, one *British Journal of Nutrition* study found that when fasting was pitted against traditional dieting, overweight women lost the same amount of bodyweight but had a greater reduction of belly fat.
- May help prevent cancer, as shown by a 2016 paper published in the journal *Metabolism in Cancer*. This may be because fasting reduces the hormone IGF-1, which is involved in the growth of cancer cells.[24-25]
- Maintain muscle while dieting. Believe it or not, some studies show that intermittent fasting is beneficial for holding on to muscle while dropping body fat. A 2011 review showed that intermittent calorie restriction caused a comparable amount of weight loss as continuous calorie restriction, *but* fat loss with the intermittent type of diet was greater, meaning subjects

maintained a greater amount of muscle mass. With traditional caloric restriction, 25 percent of the weight lost was muscle mass, whereas only 10 percent of the weight loss was muscle mass for subjects following an intermittent fasting caloric restriction diet.

- Prevent neurodegenerative disorders. Studies in animal subjects show fasting could safeguard against, and even improve outcomes for, conditions such as Alzheimer's disease and Parkinson's.

- A better night's sleep. Anecdotally, intermittent fasters report better sleep. Research is limited, but one theory is that intermittent fasting synchronizes the body's circadian rhythm, which governs sleep patterns. A regulated circadian rhythm means getting to sleep with ease and waking up well rested.

Blue Zones

Blue Zones are areas scientists have identified throughout the world where people tend to live longer and retain function with age.

Designated as a Blue Zone, Ikaria is a rustic, mountainous island in Greece where 33 percent of the population lives over the age of 90. And these folks truly live! They are not hanging on in hospice, in convalescent homes, or under any sort of medical supervision. Instead, they are vibrant, sexually active, hiking up steep trails, and enjoying life in spite of heavy wine consumption and even chain-smoking being fairly common.

How is this possible?

FASTING! As adherents of a traditional representation of Greek Orthodox Christianity, Ikarians follow a religious calendar filled with numerous holidays that include fasting as a feature of ritual and worship.

Fasting, or a calorie-restricted diet, shows up in many other long-living, healthy communities across the globe. For instance, on the island of Okinawa, which is also selected as a Blue Zone, there is a common Confucian practice of restricting calories known as *hara hachi bu*. Furthermore, until the 1960s, when many of Okinawa's current nonagenarians (people in their nineties) and centenarians (people 100 or over) were middle-aged, the far majority of Okinawans followed a traditional diet where they lived often in calorie deficit (this was before the now overwhelming presence of fast-food options on the island).

In summary, the studies and anecdotal evidence about intermittent fasting are pretty impressive. Plus, there are still many studies in progress right now, so we soon should have even more data on how intermittent fasting impacts the body. (In case you want to look the studies up, scientists usually refer to the eating style as "time-restricted eating.")

Chapter 4: Intermittent Fasting Cautions

Even though intermittent fasting is generally safe and offers numerous health benefits, you need to do what's best for you. In some situations, it's important to approach the eating style with a lot of caution or possibly avoid it. Here are four of these situations:

1. You have a blood sugar control problem

If you have diabetes or another blood sugar control issue, fasting may not be ideal since it reduces insulin levels. (On the other hand, fasting can improve insulin sensitivity, which is a good thing.)[26]

Intermittent fasting may be transformative for your health, your athletic performance, and the shape of your body. Just make sure to talk with your doctor or another medical supervisor before you start this eating style. They can help you decide whether it's right for your situation.

2. You're pregnant

There's no research on how intermittent fasting influences pregnancy. Therefore, don't try this eating style when you have a baby on the way!

Your baby needs a lot of nutrients to develop properly, and intermittent fasting may interfere with this.

3. You are underweight or have been anorexic

Since intermittent fasting tends to produce weight loss, don't follow this eating style if you're underweight or have been anorexic. You may hurt your health by losing more weight or promoting unhealthy eating habits. So, if you have had any eating disorders, avoid this style of diet.

4. Modifications for Women

Some research suggests men react better to intermittent fasting than women do. One study noted improved insulin sensitivity in men in response to fasting but worsened blood sugar control in women.[27] What's more, studies on female—but not male—rats show that long fasts may cause reproductive issues. Scientists noted fasting can cause dysregulation of the menstrual cycle and make female rats emaciated and infertile.[27-28] While there's no quality evidence available to discern whether similar adverse effects apply to humans, anecdotally, some women have noted menstrual and reproductive issues when starting intermittent fasting. Thus, if you're female, observe closely how your body responds. If you experience issues, go back to a regular eating style.

For women, we have found it works best for fasts to be between 12 and 14 hours per day. This time frame seems to prevent the downsides of intermittent fasting while providing the benefits. Always speak to your doctor before starting this style of eating regimen.

Chapter 5: How to Set Up Your Foolproof Intermittent Fasting Diet

Ready to give intermittent fasting a try? We have you covered. Follow our eight-step system to create a customized intermittent fasting plan based on what's ideal for your unique situation, goals, and preferences. You'll find out your ideal calorie and macro intake as well as how to apply that to an intermittent fasting eating style.

Step 1: Calculate your basal metabolic rate (BMR).

This stands for the number of calories you'd expend over 24 hours if you would do nothing but rest. You can calculate this number with the Harris-Benedict equation. Here's how the formula works:

- Men: (10 × weight in kg) + (6.25 × height in cm) − (5 × age in years) + 5
- Women: (10 × weight in kg) + (6.25 × height in cm) − (5 × age in years) − 161

The above is the formula revised by Mifflin and St. Jeor in 1990. It's the most accurate variant of the equation, although the formula is in metrics. If you prefer to use the imperial system, you can use the following formula:

- Men: 66 + (6.2 × weight in pounds) + (12.7 × height in inches) − (6.76 × age in years)
- Women: 655 + (4.35 × weight in pounds) + (4.7 × height in inches) − (4.7 × age in years)

For example, if you weigh 85 kilos, are 185 cm tall, and are 35 years old, the calculation would be as follows:

- Men: (10 × 85) + (6.25 × 185) − (5 × 35) + 5 = 1,836

In other words, you would burn 1,836 calories per day if you rested all day.

Step 2: Adjust your BMR to your activity level.

Commercial divers work offshore to help construct or maintain platforms for the oil and gas industry, or inland, surveying lakes and rivers for construction projects. It's a grueling profession and one that burns lots of calories—over 700 per hour! In contrast, answering phones at a call center 90 miles northeast of Nashville, Tennessee, may burn less than 100 calories per hour. Each will have different energy needs for the same goal (i.e., to get their job done).

Thus, you'll have to adjust your BMR to your activity level to figure out how many calories you burn each day. To do so, select the activity level below that best fits your situation. Make sure you are honest with yourself here because exaggerating your activity level would lead to inaccurate outcomes.

- Sedentary (e.g., no exercise and you have an office job)
- Somewhat active (e.g., you walk your dog several times a day or commute by bicycle)
- Active (e.g., you exercise regularly and are on your feet most of the day)
- Highly active (e.g., you exercise regularly and you do manual labor)

Then, apply the multiplier associated with that activity level to your BMR.

	Sedentary	Somewhat active	Active	Highly active
Male	1.0	1.12	1.27	1.54
Female	1.0	1.14	1.27	1.45

For instance, if your BMR is 1,836 and you're an active male, the math would be 1,836 x 1.27 = 2,332.

Step 3: Create a calorie deficit or surplus.

To lose body fat, you'll need to be in a calorie deficit. And to gain muscle, you'll need to be in a calorie surplus. That's why it's now time to adjust the number you calculated in the previous step to your primary fitness goal.

If you want to gain muscle, we recommend that you multiply the number by 1.15. Thus, if you ended up with 2,332 in the previous step, you would multiply that by 1.15, which means you'll get 2,682. That's the number of calories you should consume per day to gain weight and build muscle.

You can go higher than a multiple of 1.15. However, doing so will likely substantially increase the amount of fat you gain without providing much, if any, additional muscle-building benefits. That's why we recommend a calorie surplus of 15 percent as the starting point.

If your goal is to lose weight and fat, it's best to set up your calorie intake based on your current body fat percentage. That's because how much fat you carry influences whether you'll do best on a small, moderate, or large calorie deficit.

Obese and overweight people can diet aggressively, while the leaner you get, the less aggressive your approach should be. That's because if you carry many excess pounds, you aren't that prone to muscle loss on a diet. But if you are already fairly lean, it becomes more and more likely your body will burn muscle tissue as fuel when you diet.

Muscle loss is not only detrimental to your health, physical performance, and appearance, but also to your long-term fat loss results. That's because muscle is metabolically active. This means losing muscle will reduce your metabolic rate, causing you to burn fewer calories every day, which, in turn, makes it harder to lose fat and keep it off.

To determine your ideal calorie deficit, select your gender and body fat percentage from the table below. Then, apply the calorie deficit on the right to the number you calculated during the previous step.

	Body fat percentage		Calorie deficit in percentages
	Male	**Female**	
Contest prep	< 8	< 14	2.5 – 7.5
Athletic	8 – 14	14 – 24	5 – 20
Average	14 – 21	24 – 33	20 – 30
Overweight	21 – 26	33 – 39	30 – 40
Obese	> 26	> 39	40 – 50

To give you an example, let's say that you categorize as "average," that the number from your previous step is 2,332, and that you opt for a 25 percent calorie deficit. Then, you'd multiply 2,332 by 0.75, which would equal 1,749. That's the number of calories you should eat per day to optimize fat loss while minimizing muscle loss.

Please note: The calorie deficit targets above are a guideline. We don't recommend that you take a more aggressive approach because that would increase muscle wasting. However, you can take a slower approach, if you want. Some people find that a slower approach is more achievable and/or makes it easier to adhere to their plan. The downside is that a smaller calorie deficit would increase the time it'll take to reach your goal. So, that's something to consider, based on your preferences.

Step 4: Track your calories.

Yes, it's vital to keep track of your calories because people underestimate how many calories they take in by up to 45 percent.[29] That's why it's very likely that you don't consume the right number of calories, if you don't keep track. And, when you miscalculate your calories, you may compromise your results.

Additionally, research also shows that keeping track of your calories improves results. For instance, one meta-analysis found that weight loss programs involving calorie tracking produce, on average, 3.3 kilograms more weight loss over one year than those that don't.[30]

For muscle growth, you'll also see better results when you track your calories. That's because doing so will help you ensure that you obtain the recommended 15 percent calorie surplus. If you don't keep track, you may consume more than that, which would increase fat storage. Or if you consume less, you would impair muscle growth.

Keep in mind:

- Protein provides 4 calories per gram
- Carbs provide 4 calories per gram
- Dietary fat provides 9 calories per gram
- Alcohol provides 7 calories per gram

We advise abstaining from alcohol altogether or having one to two drinks a week, at the most.

Fortunately, it doesn't have to take a lot of time to track your caloric intake. That's because apps such as MyFitnessPal and Cronometer can do the math for you. All you have to do is enter the foods you eat, and the software will show you how many calories you ate as well as from which macronutrients these calories came.

Step 5: Determine your macros.

It's important to ensure that you get your calories from the right macros, which refers to your intake of protein, carbs, and dietary fat.

Protein is the most important of those macronutrients because it aids muscle growth, fat loss, and gym performance. It's the building block of muscle, which is why getting enough of it benefits muscle growth in a calorie surplus and prevents muscle loss during a cut.

Besides, protein is the most satiating macronutrient. An adequate intake supports weight loss by reducing hunger, as shown by research published in the *American Journal of Clinical Nutrition*.[31]

In the study, subjects raised their protein intake from 15 percent to 30 percent of their daily caloric consumption. As a result, they consumed, on average, 441 fewer calories per day, which led to an average weight loss of 11 pounds in 12 weeks—just by eating more protein!

The question is: How much protein do you need? You should opt for one gram per pound of bodyweight per day. So, if you weigh 187 pounds (85 kg), that would be at least 187 grams of protein daily. You can go above that amount, but it won't enhance your results further. Thus, you could also get extra calories in the form of carbs or dietary fat. Since protein provides four calories per gram, this means 748 of your calories should come from protein (187 x 4 =748).

Once you know your daily protein target, get the rest of your calories from carbs and fat. We've bundled these two together because the ratio between them isn't that important for body composition. Generally, though, it's best to consume carbs and fat in a balanced fashion. You do that by eating a broad spectrum of healthy foods like fish, meat, eggs, dairy, nuts, seeds, fruit, and vegetables.

Citing the previous example, if you weigh 85 kilos, are 185 cm tall, and are 35 years old, the calculation would be as follows:

- BMR for men: $(10 \times 85) + (6.25 \times 185) - (5 \times 35) + 5 = 1,836$

In other words, you would burn 1,836 calories per day if you rested all day. To adjust for activity level, if you're an active male with a BMR of 1,836, the math would be 1,836 x 1.27 = 2,332. Now let's suppose you are 17 percent body fat, and you want to reduce body fat from here.

If you opt for a 25 percent calorie deficit, you'd calculate (2,332 x .75) = 1,749 calories per day.

You will get 748 of those calories from protein (187 x 4.) The remaining 1,001 calories will come from fat and carbohydrates (1749 – 748 = 1,001.)

A good place to start is equally splitting carbohydrates and fat, so this would mean 500 grams of each (1,001/2 = 500.5.)

This would mean you eat 56 grams of fat per day, since (500/9) = 55.55. (Remember a fat gram has 9 calories.)

This would also mean you consume 125 grams of carbohydrates (500/4) = 125.

Your daily total would be 187 grams of protein, 56 grams of fat, and 125 grams of carbs. Start with equal caloric amounts of carbs and fat, then adjust from there; the key is calories in verses calories out as long as protein requirements are being met.

If you act on that and make sure you get enough calories and protein, your carb and fat intakes tend to take care of themselves. You'll get enough carbs to aid workout performance. And you'll get enough dietary fat to support hormone production and general health.

Now, there are two exceptions. If you're a woman with polycystic ovary syndrome (PCOS) or you have impaired insulin sensitivity (e.g., due to excess body weight), a lower-carb, higher-fat approach may be beneficial. That's because in such cases, you may get better fat loss, muscle growth, and health outcomes by cutting carbs and eating more fat.[32-35] As always, we strongly recommend talking with your doctor before changing your eating plan.

The bottom line is this: Both higher-carb, low-fat diets and low-carb, high-fat diets can work for fat loss, and this has been demonstrated over and over in research. So long as calories and protein intake are controlled, it really doesn't matter which diet an individual follows—at the end of the day it's calories in versus calories out.

Step 6: Decide on your intermittent fasting style.

While there are many different forms of effective intermittent fasting, the one we recommend is the 16:8 method. We give this recommendation for two reasons:

1. Fasting for longer than 16 hours per day, which some styles have you do, may cause muscle wasting (or, in case you want to build muscle, prevent you from gaining the greatest amount of mass possible).
2. Many intermittent fasting diets (including 5:2 and Eat-Stop-Eat) promote an irregular daily eating pattern. That can impair insulin sensitivity and metabolic rate, worsen heart health, and increase hunger.[35-41]

Here's how you execute the 16:8 method:

If you're male, fast for 16 hours per day and eat your foods in a daily feeding window of 8 hours. If you're female, fast for 12 to 14 hours per day and eat your foods in a daily feeding window of 10 to 12 hours.

During your fast, don't consume any calories. What you do want to consume are non-caloric fluids like water, tea, and black coffee.

It's essential to drink a lot because you're more prone to dehydration during a fast. Drink a minimum of half an ounce of water per pound of bodyweight daily. You want to focus on drinking lots of water because you normally get much of your hydration through food. So, you want to compensate for the water you're not receiving from food.

It's best to fast in the morning and consume most of your calories in the afternoon and evening. There are a number of reasons for that.

First, it tends to be harder to control calorie intake by eating in the morning and fasting in the evening. That's because the natural appetite of most people peaks at around 8:00 p.m.[36]

Second, eating in the evening aids sleep quality. It does so by activating the parasympathetic "rest and digest" state. (That's why people often become tired after a meal.)

Third, social meals and activities with food are much more likely in the evening. Just because you are following an intermittent fast does not mean that you have to convert to living like an ascetic recluse. While the life of a hermit has many valuable aspects, it is important for social, emotional, and intellectual health to maintain a healthy social life. This style of intermittent fasting allows you to do that.

As an added benefit, not eating early in the day prevents the activation of the parasympathetic state (this is when the body is relaxed, resting, and/or feeding). While this is a desirable place when you're kicking back on a folding chair at the beach, this is not where you want to be when you need to do your job, train hard, and get through your day. By not eating early in the day, you keep yourself from entering this state. The result is that you'll feel more energized, ready to tackle whatever your day brings.

One way you could set up your nutrition pattern is by eating between 1 p.m. and 9 p.m. and fasting for the rest of the time. How you set up the exact hours is up to you, but try to maintain consistency.

During your eating window, focus on hitting your calorie and macronutrient targets. That ensures you'll indeed progress toward your fat loss and muscle building goals.

Step 7: Stay consistent.

Irregular meal patterns have adverse physiological effects. They disrupt postprandial metabolism, which means they cause your body to react to food less well.

Here are the adverse effects of an irregular meal pattern:

- Worsened cardiovascular health due to increased blood pressure and higher levels of total and LDL ("bad") cholesterol.[37-38]
- Higher risk of overeating and fat gain due to increased hunger levels and reduced satisfaction from eating.[39-40]
- Lowered thermic effect of food, which means a reduced metabolic rate.[41]
- Decreased insulin sensitivity after your meal, which is unfavorable for fat burning and health.[42]

So, pick a particular meal frequency; for example, eat four times per day. Then decide at which time you'll eat those meals and stick to it every day.

Such consistency can be hard at times, especially due to social activities, but make your best effort to follow through. One tip that can help here is to set the alarm on your phone for when it's time to eat.

Also, the fact that it's beneficial to be consistent doesn't mean you can't follow an intermittent fasting eating style—you can. However, make sure to follow a similar protocol every day of the week. For example, don't fast for 16 hours today, for 14 hours tomorrow, and for 18 hours the day after. Instead, pick a particular method and maintain it.

Step 8: Make the right food choices.

Go on Instagram and you will see the IIFYM (If It Fits Your Macros) cult proselytizing their methodology with pictures of carefully weighed and measured tilapia with exactly 1.4 Ding Dongs.

Here are examples of two diets. Both contain roughly 2,300 calories. Diet One is made up of calorie-dense foods and thus would not be ideal for weight loss. Diet Two contains low-energy but highly satiating foods and is an example of a proper fat-loss diet.

Diet One:

Meal	Food + serving	Calories
#1	McDonald's Big Mac (one serving)	541
#1	Coca-Cola (one large bottle)	273
#2	French fries (300 grams)	471
#2	Mayonnaise (2 tbsp)	280
#3	Chicken nuggets (150 grams)	465
#3	Vanilla ice cream (100 grams)	310
Total number of calories: 2,340		

Diet Two:

Meal	Food + serving	Calories
#1	Eggs, whole, hard-cooked (3 medium)	205
#1	Apple, fresh, with skin (1 medium)	95
#1	Greek yogurt, plain, nonfat with fresh blueberries (300 grams + 75 grams)	220
#1	Coffee, prepared from grounds	5
#2	Caesar salad with shrimp (300 grams)	313
#2	Avocado, Hass (1 medium)	227
#2	Strawberries, raw (250 grams)	80

	Salmon (200 grams)	364
	Green beans (200 grams)	70
#3	Boiled potatoes (200 grams)	152
	Lemon (1 medium)	17
	Crème fraîche, reduced-fat (200 grams)	326
#4	Whey protein shake (1 scoop of 31 grams)	124
	Banana (1 medium)	105
Total number of calories: 2,303		

Proper food selection is vital for the following reasons:

First, certain foods are more filling than others. And if you mostly consume satiating foods, you'll suffer fewer cravings, and thus it'll be easier to keep your calorie intake under control.

For example, even though croissants contain five times more calories than boiled potatoes, the latter was found to be seven times more satiating. In other words, it'll be much easier to obtain and maintain a healthy weight if you get your calories from boiled potatoes than from croissants.

Second, the amount of vitamins, minerals, trace minerals, and other beneficial compounds varies among foods. This matters because most of these compounds influence bodily functions related to your figure and athletic performance, such as hormone and energy production and fat oxidation.

Third, certain foods are more beneficial for health than others. Now, if you mainly eat these healthy foods, you'll feel more vigorous and vital. As a result, you'll have more energy and motivation to go to the gym, stick to your diet, and still be up for an active "personal life."

Moreover, maintaining a healthy diet will reduce your chance of getting sick. This is important because if you're sick, you can't work out (at least not optimally). Missing your workouts or training at a lower level may reduce your progress and cause you to lose your gains, especially if you're sick over a long time frame.

How to Optimize Food Selection

When you're shopping for food at the market, one applicable approach to healthy food selection is to stay on the perimeter (in other words, avoid aisles filled with the processed, sugar-heavy options). This will allow you to select foods that are filled with your daily nutrients and support your fitness goals. Remember to get at least 80 percent of your foods from whole, nutritious sources such as fruits, vegetables, meat, fish, nuts, seeds, and healthy oils. Consume a bare minimum of four servings of fruits and vegetables a day and shoot for more than five. In addition, maintain a varied diet so that you get a wide range of nutrients.

Focusing on nutrient-dense, low-calorie foods is especially important on a fat-loss diet because it aids hunger control, making it easier to maintain your calorie target. When your goal is dropping body fat, get your protein intake by consuming primarily lean protein sources like chicken and tuna. This helps to keep your calorie intake in control. In addition, avoid starchy carbs such as white rice and bread because they provide many calories without satiating hunger effectively.

When you're on a muscle-building diet, you should still consume primarily nutrient-dense foods. However, since gaining weight requires an increased calorie intake, it's okay to consume more energy-dense foods (as long as you don't overreach your calorie target). Remember, even if you're looking to gain weight, if the cashier at your local chain fast-food spot knows you by name, this is an indication that you should dial back on the junk food.

Examples of energy-dense foods are starchy carbs (rice, quinoa, oatmeal, etc.), fattier cuts of meat (beef, pork, lamb), higher-fat dairy (full-fat milk, full-fat yogurt, cheese, etc.), and nuts and seeds. Adding those foods into your diet is especially helpful if you have difficulty consuming enough calories.

To make sure that you get enough of each vitamin and mineral, it is best to get a blood panel test done to evaluate your levels of each micronutrient. But since that may be pricey and inconvenient, an alternative is tracking your food intake with the app Cronometer (www.cronometer.com). If you log your food into the app, it automatically calculates your intake of essential vitamins and minerals.

Now, if it turns out that you regularly consume too little of a specific micronutrient, then adjust your intake accordingly. Just search online for foods that are rich in that particular nutrient and add one or more of them into your diet. For example, if your zinc intake is subpar, then consuming oysters, lamb, or pumpkin seeds can offer the solution. Also, taking the nutrient in supplement form or consuming a high-quality multivitamin is beneficial for reaching your daily nutritional needs.

Chapter 6: The Pros and Cons of Longer Fasts

In general, we recommend the 16:8 intermittent fasting method, which means you fast for 16 hours per day and eat your foods in an 8-hour feeding window. However, depending on your situation and goals, you may also want to do a longer fast occasionally, such as by going without food for 48 hours.

The main benefit of a longer fast is that it increases autophagy, a word derived from the Greek *auto* (self) and *phagein* (to eat). Thus, autophagy is the body's way of cleaning out damaged cells to regenerate newer and healthier ones.

It's beyond the scope of this book to explain the specifics of how autophagy works. And even scientists are still trying to figure it out. But in a broad sense, autophagy drops when insulin and amino acid levels rise. And autophagy increases when insulin and amino acid levels drop.[43]

Now, the thing with longer fasts is that they produce a more significant reduction in insulin and amino acid levels, which makes them superior for stimulating autophagy.

Unfortunately, scientists don't yet know how to measure autophagy in humans directly. Instead, they look at various blood markers associated with autophagy, which is quite unreliable, making it hard to draw conclusions. However, animal research shows that long-term fasts may be beneficial.

For example, in a study from the Keio University Graduate School of Pharmaceutical Sciences, researchers gave mice either unlimited access to food or starved them for two days. Then, they euthanized all the mice and collected blood and tissue samples to measure autophagy markers.

The result? The mice that hadn't eaten had significantly higher autophagy markers. Sure, this study was done on mice, and it's unclear whether the same results apply to humans. But many leading experts on fasting believe that they do.

Thus, if you want to use fasting to improve your health and well-being, you may want to consider doing longer-term fasts, such as going without food for 48 hours. The autophagy benefits may enhance your health in many ways.

Besides stimulating autophagy, another benefit of doing a longer fast is that it can put you into a deep state of ketosis. We've covered in detail what ketosis is and why it is beneficial in our book *Keto Built*, so if you want to learn more, check it out. But to highlight some of the benefits, ketosis supports fat loss (especially around the midsection) as well as heart and brain health.

Something to keep in mind, however, is that after fasting for about 20 hours mTOR signaling (which regulates cell metabolism, growth, proliferation, and survival) decreases.[44] The mTOR pathway is important for muscle growth and maintenance, which is one reason extended fasts may promote muscle wasting. That's why we don't recommend that you do an extended fast often.

However, if you're up for the challenge and want to enjoy the potential benefits of autophagy, you should consider doing a 48-hour fast once every quarter or even yearly, if you are not doing our adapted ketogenic fast.

Let's take a look at what happens in longer fasts.

24-48 hours: The liver begins producing glucose from amino acids in a process called gluconeogenesis; this is the same process we wrote about in *Keto Built* as occurring when ketogenic diets consist of excessive amounts of protein.

48-72 hours: At this point, the liver's energy has been totally depleted and ketosis is initiated. Here, the body begins to break down fat for energy; the fat is broken down to produce ketones, which are used by the brain for energy.

Beyond 72 hours: Advocates point out the high level of growth hormone stimulation that might help preserve muscle mass; the idea is that fatty acids and ketones deliver energy, and the increase in adrenaline prevents a drastic drop in metabolism. For longer fasts, we recommend checking out Elliott Hulse's ebook, *Rational Fasting*.

Our adapted ketogenic fast (AKF) has been our most successful fasting fat-loss plan. The results have been astounding.

Adapted Ketogenic Fast

A ketogenic diet is low in carbs, high in fat, and moderate in protein. Dietary fats replace the majority of carbs you cut and deliver approximately 75 percent of your total calorie intake.

A critical mistake dieters frequently make is consuming excessive protein, so, at best, they achieve a state of gluconeogenesis. The reality is, protein should account for approximately 20 percent of your caloric intake and carbs should be 5 percent of your daily intake.

Reducing carbs to this level forces your body to rely on fats for its main energy source instead of glucose.

In ketosis, your body uses ketones—molecules produced in your liver from fats when glucose is limited.

Traditional nutritionists advocate avoiding fat like the plague because of its high calorie content, but both research and anecdotal evidence show that ketogenic diets are superior at shredding body fat compared to low-fat diets.

An added bonus is that a ketogenic diet reduces hunger and increases satiety.

Ideally, a ketogenic diet should consist of eggs, meat, poultry, full-fat dairy, nuts, full-fat cheese, nut butter, fatty fish, olive oil, coconut oil, avocado oil, sesame oil, avocados, non-starchy vegetables, and condiments that do not contain carbohydrates.

Combining the ketogenic diet with intermittent fasting often produces a synergistic fat-loss effect.

The Plan

Ultimately, fat loss is achieved via calories in versus calories out; so, even if you're fasting, if you consume as much as and whatever the hell you want, you will not lose body fat if this puts you over your daily calorie expenditure. Throughout this plan, in all phases, we recommend drinking a minimum of half an ounce of water per pound of bodyweight daily, and ideally closer to 1.5 times your bodyweight in pounds. A 200-pound person will ideally drink 300 or more ounces of water a day.

Initiation Phase: To begin on our keto fasting plan, for two and a half days, you are going to do a complete fast. You can consume water, black coffee, or green tea; caffeinated beverages are fine as long as they are calorie-free, but we do advise avoiding artificial sweeteners, with the exception of stevia. Co-author Josh Bryant has pushed this phase up to five days with success, but we recommend sticking with two and a half days. For example, have your last meal Monday evening and end the initiation phase Thursday morning.

Fasting Ketogenic Bliss Phase: After the initiation, follow the caloric fat-loss formula (found in chapter 5) to figure out your caloric needs; this is your baseline. Continue for a minimum of 14 days and a maximum of 42 days; we recommend 21 days as a starting point.

You have an eight-hour feeding window during this phase; you can shorten this if you want, but do not increase it. All calories must be consumed within the eight hours. Most people will have no need to shorten this window.

During this phase, a sample meal plan looks like the following:

10 a.m. Breakfast Black coffee with 1 ounce (oz) of grass-fed whipping cream, 3 scrambled eggs topped with avocado slices

1 p.m. Lunch Large, leafy green salad topped with 2 tablespoons (tbsp) of olive oil, vinegar, and 3 oz fatty salmon cooked in grass-fed bacon fat, sprinkled with three crumbled slices of bacon

3 p.m. Snack (optional) 1/2 cup Brazil nuts

6 p.m. Dinner 8 oz rib-eye and 2 cups of asparagus topped with 2 tbsp of grass-fed butter

You can have as few or as many meals as you want during this eight-hour period, as long as you don't exceed your caloric intake target.

Refeed Day: After you've completed the Fasting Ketogenic Bliss Phase, you get a day with no rules! Now, for health purposes and so you don't have to camp out on the toilet for days on end, we recommend doubling your caloric intake, so if you've been consuming 2,100 calories, that total becomes 4,200 calories. At least 50 percent of those calories should come from carbohydrates.

Some of the best carb sources for a refeed:

- Starchy vegetables such as potatoes, squash, yams, etc.
- Grains like white rice, quinoa, oats, etc.
- Whole fruits
- Nutritive sweeteners such as honey, maple syrup, or blackstrap molasses

Here is a sample refeed day:

Breakfast: 4 whole wheat pancakes with maple syrup, 1 scoop of whey protein powder

Snack: 10 oz of yam topped with 1/2 cup of raspberries

Lunch: Large turkey sandwich on whole grain bread with tomatoes, lettuce, and mustard, two pieces of fruit

Snack: Shake made with cow's or plant-based milk, bananas, berries, hemp seeds, and whey protein powder

Dinner: 4 tuna rolls, 2 large dragon fruits

Dessert: 1/2 cup of chocolate pudding

Admittedly, most people do whatever the hell they want on their refeed day and it becomes a cheat day. Usually, there's no adverse effects to fat loss, and at most it results in a mildly upset stomach. These folks feel the trade-off is worth the fun, and some believe this metabolic shock further intensifies fat loss.

An example of a free-for-all cheat day could look like the following:

Breakfast: Waffle House All-Star Special, double waffle, triple hash browns
Lunch: Medium peperoni pizza, Caesar salad
Dinner: Sushi buffet, 1 sake, 2 Asahi beers
Dessert: Braum's triple-dip sundae with caramel and no nuts

After the refeed day, the cycle starts over with the initiation phase and you repeat the process. This should be done a minimum of three times and a maximum of ten times over a six month period.

Chapter 7: Frequently Asked Questions

Q: What can I drink during my fast?

All calorie-free drinks, such as water, tea, and black coffee. While we don't recommend diet sodas because of the artificial sweeteners they contain, many people have successfully dropped body fat drinking diet sodas during a fast. Studies suggest they don't raise insulin or blood sugar, which means they don't break your fast.[43-45] And other evidence suggests zero-calorie sweeteners are safe as long as they are consumed in moderation.[46-48]

Q: How much should I drink during my fast?

More than what you would normally drink. That's because your hydration needs are higher during a fast. One reason is that fasting reduces insulin levels, which causes your kidneys to secrete sodium and water from the body.[49-50] Besides, most fluids are generally consumed during a meal, and since you don't eat during a fast, you'll have to compensate for this by drinking more.[51-52]

Remember that your body is made up of around 60 to 70 percent water. This water is present in all your cells, organs, and tissues to support proper functioning and temperature regulation. In other words, water is crucial for surviving, let alone thriving. The problem? Most of us are chronically dehydrated. While it's hard to put a figure on dehydration prevalence, a survey of 3,003 Americans found that 75 percent likely had a net fluid loss, leading to chronic dehydration. Such a lack of bodily fluids can have severe side effects, not only on your health but also on your athletic performance and how you look in the buff.

Astonishingly, those who don't habitually drink water consume, on average, 9 percent more calories daily than those who do. For an average adult male, that represents around 1,575 more calories a week (based on an energy need of 2,500 calories), which, energy-wise, equals roughly 0.45 pound of pure fat. The reason why dehydration increases calorie intake—and thereby raises the risk of weight and fat gain—is that your brain can't effectively distinguish the difference between thirst and hunger. So being dehydrated may cause you to reach for a meal even though what you need is a glass of water.

But that's not all! Dehydration also hampers athletic performance. Mild dehydration of just 3 to 4 percent of body mass loss reduces strength by around 2 percent (that's roughly 12 pounds off a 600-pound deadlift), and more severe dehydration lowers performance even further. Dehydration impairs performance because it reduces motivation, raises fatigue, alters body temperature control, and makes exercise feel a lot harder, both physically and mentally. The result? Because you won't be able to train optimally in the gym, you can't maximally stimulate your muscles, which leads to diminished progress.

Staying hydrated is also crucial for muscle growth. One reason for this is that muscles are made up of about 75 to 80 percent water. That's why a hydrated muscle looks fuller and larger compared to a dehydrated one. Plus, research also shows that muscle cell hydration status influences protein synthesis and breakdown rates. In other words, getting enough water aids muscle growth.

How to Calculate Your Daily Water Intake Needs

Generally, we recommend ½ ounce of water for every pound in body-weight. Yet, there's no set-in-stone number on optimal water intake, because we all have different fluid intake needs due to various factors such as body size, activity levels, and the environment we're in. That's why it's not ideal to aim to consume a specified amount of water each day. Instead, to figure out how much water you should drink for optimal health and fitness progress, it's better to evaluate your urination habits. This allows you to see if you're getting enough water. How do you do this? It's simple. Aim for at least five clear urinations a day. That is five urinations during which your urine is clear; not five in total!

You want your urine to be clear and copious, at least five times daily. If you accomplish that, you're well-hydrated. If not, you need to consume more water.

If you're not getting enough water daily, one excellent way to raise your intake of it is to consume one glass of water before each meal. So if you eat four meals per day, for example, that would raise your daily water intake by around 800 milliliters. But besides raising your water intake, drinking a glass of water before your meal also has another benefit: It can increase feelings of fullness and thereby reduce your total calorie intake. This is because water consumption causes your stomach wall to stretch, which signals to your brain that your stomach is fuller. For example, one study on obese older adults found that drinking 500 milliliters of water 30 minutes before breakfast decreased calorie consumption by an average of 13 percent.

Q: How can I manage hunger during a fast?

First, keep in mind that the hunger tends to be severe only during the first few days (if at all). Once your body has adapted to the new eating schedule, you'll suffer significantly fewer cravings.

Still, aside from giving your body time to get used to fasting, there are some things you can do. The main one is to ensure you stay well-hydrated. That's important because the brain isn't that good at distinguishing the difference between hunger and thirst. As a result, what we interpret as hunger cravings are often caused by dehydration instead of a need for food.

It may be especially beneficial to drink coffee. Many people find that coffee helps them control hunger better during a fast. Ideally, though, don't drink too much coffee after 1 p.m. to ensure the caffeine won't interfere with your sleep.

Speaking of sleep, not getting enough of it is another common reason for hunger cravings. Research shows that poor sleep lowers satiating hormones like leptin while raising the hunger hormone ghrelin.[52] Thus, get enough sleep. It'll help you control cravings. Plus, it also benefits health and body composition.

Q: Can I take supplements while fasting?

Yes, you can. However, do keep in mind that some compounds are best absorbed when consumed alongside dietary fat. The fat-soluble vitamins D and K are two examples.

Five supplements to consider are the following: magnesium, vitamin D, multivitamins, citrulline, and caffeine.

Q: Can I work out while I'm fasting?

Yes, fasted workouts are fine, although you may want to consume 10 milligrams of branched-chain amino acids (BCAAs) before your session. That'll help you reduce muscle wasting while interfering with your fast only minimally.

Some even classify fasted workouts as a multi-therapeutic approach because you derive the synergy of both the exercise and fasting benefits. They potentially boost each other's benefits to a level that exceeds that of each combined.

An effective way to implement this strategy is to train prior to your first meal of the day. Training too late at night can throw off the body's natural circadian rhythm.

Q: How would you work intermittent fasting around training?

The fast we recommend is 16 hours with an 8-hour feeding window. With this as a framework, let's say you plan your workout during your lunch break at noon. Here is how your workout, fasting, and eating could look.

6:00 a.m. Wake up

8:00 a.m. Arrive at work

12:00 p.m. Training (bodybuilding leg workout: squats, leg presses, leg curls, Romanian deadlifts, bodyweight finisher)

1:00 p.m. Meal 1 (Post Workout): 2 slices of Ezekiel Bread French toast with 2 tbsp of maple syrup, 5 whole eggs, 5 egg whites, 1 piece of fruit

4:30 p.m.   Meal 2: 10 oz sirloin steak, 2 cups of sautéed vegetables, 1 medium sweet potato, 1 cup of berries

7:30 p.m.   Meal 3: 8 oz tilapia, medium Caesar salad, 2 protein brownies

After employing intermittent fasting, many find that they like to work out fasted! We recommend you have a meal post workout. So, following this model, you could also work out later in the afternoon or evening and have your post-workout meal at 4:30 or 7:30 p.m.

Q: What about alcohol consumption?

To look better in that spring break beach pic and to perform your best in athletic pursuits or during modern "courting rituals," it's best to avoid alcohol. Alcohol impairs fat burning, increases fat storage, and raises nitrogen excretion. The latter means that it hampers muscle mass; it makes you more prone to muscle loss on a weight-loss diet and impairs growth on a mass-gaining plan.

That said, most people like to have a drink—and then some—once in a while. If that's you, then you may be wondering how to drink alcohol without derailing your fitness progress. Well, good news! There are a few things you can do to minimize the negative effects of alcohol (on your fitness goals, that is; not necessarily on your health, your relationships, and your odd tendency to wake up disrobed on your neighbor's front lawn after "tying one on").

First, limit your relationship with alcohol to moderate consumption up to twice a week at most. Ideally, this would be on a day that you don't work out, to reduce the negative effects alcohol has on recovery and muscle growth. Second, track the macros that are in your beverages, and count alcoholic calories toward your carb intake. Third, try to limit alcohol consumption to at most two drinks. However, even though it's not ideal, it's okay to go over this amount once in a while, if you still hit your macros and don't make it a habit.

The bottom line is power drinking impairs power building.

Q: Is it unhealthy to skip breakfast?

Some studies do show that breakfast skippers are generally less healthy than those who eat breakfast regularly. However, that's not because there is anything inherently bad about skipping breakfast. Instead, it is because those who skip breakfast also tend to lead an unhealthy lifestyle, often including inactivity, smoking, and other detrimental behaviors.

If you practice intermittent fasting properly, it is not bad to skip breakfast but can even be beneficial. To learn more about this, please revisit chapter 2.

Q: Won't vitamins adversely affect the fast?

No, they won't because they don't have an acute effect on insulin levels.

Q: Does fasting slow down my metabolism?

No. Better yet, short-term fasts boost metabolism by 3.6 percent to 14 percent.[1-2]

Q: What about refeeds?

There is a time and a place!

How to use refeeds: If you are on a fat-loss plan, use refeeds to boost your results. How often you do a refeed depends on your body fat percentage. If you are a man at or above 15 percent body fat or a woman at or above 23 percent body fat, refeed once every 14 days. If you are a man with a body fat percentage below 15 percent or a woman below 23 percent body fat, refeed once every seven days. You want to refeed more often as you get leaner because you are more prone to dieting-induced adaptations. It is important that you plan in advance the day and time you will do this refeed.

On your refeed day, raise your calorie intake by 30 percent above your regular consumption. So, if you are dieting on 2,100 calories a day, consume 2,730 calories during your refeed. Whether you spread those extra calories out over the day or take them all at one sitting is up to you. Both are fine, although most people note that consuming all the extra calories in one meal is most satiating. That is, one trip to your favorite local all-you-can-eat can be cathartic on both a nutritional and emotional level.

When it comes to your macro intake during your refeed, here is what to do: First, consume between 0.81 and 1.22 grams of protein per pound of bodyweight. Second, keep your dietary fat intake below 60 grams. Do this because dietary fat isn't effective at raising the satiating hormone leptin—one of the main goals of doing a refeed—and because this macro is most likely to be stored as body fat during a refeed.

Third, minimize alcohol consumption as this macro inhibits leptin. If you want to consume an alcoholic beverage, go for one standard-size drink at most and count the calories toward your total energy intake. Fourth, get the remainder of your calories from carbs. You want to do this for the following three reasons: This macro most significantly raises leptin levels; it refills muscle glycogen stores (which naturally decline on a weight-loss plan) and thereby aids workout performance; and this macro is least likely to be stored as body fat during a refeed.

Keep the following in mind with refeeds:

- If you're on a weight-loss plan, your body will adapt to prevent you from losing too much weight too fast. It does this by downregulating metabolism, raising hunger levels, and reducing motivation to work out and move.
- These bodily changes make it harder and harder to lose weight once you get leaner.
- Doing diet breaks and refeeds will reduce the severity of these adaptations.
- On a weight-loss plan, do a diet break once every 8 to 10 weeks of calorie-restricted dieting according to the guidelines above (chapter 6).
- On a weight-loss plan, do a refeed once every 14 days if you're a man at or above 15 percent body fat or a woman at or above 23 percent, and once every 7 days if you are a man with a

body fat percentage below 15 percent or a woman below 23 percent body fat, according to the guideline above.

Q: What about nutrient timing?

Post-workout: If you consumed protein before your session, you don't need to consume post-workout nutrients as soon as possible. It takes a few hours before the nutrients from a meal reach your bloodstream, so you'll have enough amino acids floating through your veins, ready to be taken up by the cells in your muscles. The same holds true for consuming carbs immediately after your session—it's not necessary for optimal recovery and growth (although there's nothing wrong with it either if your macros allow it). An exception is if you worked out strenuously for more than an hour. In such a case, a fast-acting protein source such as whey can be beneficial.

Pre-bed: Consuming protein before going to sleep can be beneficial because it aids muscle growth. Besides, you may also want to consume some of your daily carb intake a few hours before hitting the sack. Doing so raises serotonin levels in your brain, which helps you fall asleep more quickly. As a side note, this is why we recommend cheat meals or refeeds at night. Also, some dietary fat is okay as it helps with stabilizing blood sugar levels, which makes you less likely to wake up in the middle of the night. In other words, consume a protein-rich, balanced meal a few hours before going to bed.

Q: What about carb cycling with intermittent fasting?

Carb cycling is a popular eating style among lifters. It is based on consuming more carbs but less dietary fat on workout days, and doing the opposite on days you rest (fewer carbs, more dietary fat). A favorite among bodybuilding and fat-loss coaches, the idea behind carb cycling is that it expedites fat loss and muscle growth due to its effect on insulin. In a nutshell, the increased carb intake on workout days raises insulin levels, which is thought to aid muscle growth. On the other hand, the reduced carb intake on rest days lowers insulin, which should enhance fat burning since insulin impairs fat burning (what's known as antilipolytic).

Although there's no hard research on this eating style, it would be irresponsible to completely dismiss it. The bottom line is that following carb cycling won't impede your results, and it potentially will give you a slight boost in performance. It could even help you look better naked.

While there are different approaches to carb cycling, here's what we recommend you do: Split up your weekly macro intake between high-carb and low-carb days. Then, on workout days, consume most of your calories (protein excluded) from carbs and limit your intake of dietary fat to at most 60 grams. And on rest days, limit your carb intake to at most 100 grams and get the majority of your calories from dietary fat. As long as you stick to your fasting window and your caloric requirements, by all means give this methodology a shot!

Q: What about borrowing calories?

Borrowing refers to eating slightly more on one day and somewhat less on another, while still hitting your calorie intake goal on a weekly basis. So, let's say that you overate by 300 calories on Monday. In such a case, you can reduce your energy consumption on Tuesday by 300 calories to make up for it. By doing this, you'll still hit your calorie target in the grand scheme of things.

Easy, right? But there are a few crucial things to keep in mind when borrowing. First, avoid raising or lowering your calorie intake by more than 20 percent a day. So, if 2,000 is your daily energy target, don't borrow more than 400 calories on any given day. Second, don't use the concept of borrowing as an excuse to slack on your diet. Rather, use borrowing only when it's impossible or very impractical to stay consistent with your diet that day!

Here is the bottom line: When you start to exceed the 20 percent range, you are no longer borrowing. You are overhauling. Actions have consequences. If you overhaul your daily target calorie count too much or too often, you may be purchasing a ticket to Fat Camp in Soft City (while not a desirable destination, it is a popular one). This strategy of borrowing is for special occasions and unforeseen circumstances, not because you are embarrassed to pop out Tupperware at a lunch meeting or your manager is making Grandma's dumpling recipe.

Q: Does fasting deprive your body of nutrients?

As stated earlier, you can take vitamins on your fast. And if you have body fat beyond 4 percent, you have undigested foods hanging on your insides. In a fasted state, the body will syphon nutrients from the undigested food to help meet its needs.

Q: On fasts do people feel anxiety and get headaches?

Initially some do, yes. But remember hunger is not cumulative! This could be your body detoxing, withdrawing from an emotional food addiction, withdrawing from sugar, or just the fulfillment of a self-ful-filling prophecy. Once the mental barrier is broken and you fast more frequently, you will feel better.

References

1. Mansell, P. I., Fellows, I. W., & Macdonald, I. A. (1990). Enhanced thermogenic response to epinephrine after 48-h starvation in humans. *American Journal of Physiology, 258*(1;2), 87-93.
2. Zauner, C., Schneeweiss, B., Kranz, A., Madl, C., Ratheiser, K., Kramer, L., … Lenz, K. (2000). Resting energy expenditure in short-term starvation is increased as a result of an increase in serum nor-epinephrine. *American Journal of Clinical Nutrition, 71*(6), 1511-5.
3. Ho, K. Y., Veldhuis, J. D., Johnson, M. L., Furlanetto, R., Evans, W. S., Alberti, K. G., & Thorner, M. O. (1988). Fasting enhances growth hormone secretion and amplifies the complex rhythms of growth hormone secretion in man. *Journal of Clinical Investigation, 81*(4), 968-75.
4. Heilbronn, L. K., Smith, S. R., Martin, C. K., Anton, S. D., & Ravussin, E. (2005). Alternate-day fasting in nonobese subjects: Effects on body weight, body composition, and energy metabolism. *American Journal of Clinical Nutrition, 81*(1), 69-73.
5. Ludwig, D. S., & Friedman, M. I. (2014). Increasing adiposity: Consequence or cause of overeating? *JAMA, 311*(21), 2167-8.
6. Lustig, R. H. (2006). Childhood obesity: Behavioral aberration or biochemical drive? Reinterpreting the First Law of Thermodynamics. *Nature Clinical Practice Endocrinology & Metabolism, 2*(8), 447-58.
7. Zauner, C., Schneeweiss, B., Kranz, A., Madl, C., Ratheiser, K., Kramer, L., … Lenz, K. (2000). Resting energy expenditure in short-term starvation is increased as a result of an increase in serum nor-epinephrine. *The American Journal of Clinical Nutrition, 71*(6), 1511-5.
8. Gonzalez, J. T., Veasey, R. C., Fumbold, P. L., & Stevenson, E. J. (2013). Breakfast and exercise contingently affect postprandial metabolism and energy balance in physically active males. *British Journal of Nutrition, 110*(4), 721-32.

9. Levitsky, D. A., & Pacanowski, C. R. (2013). Effect of skipping break-fast on subsequent energy intake. *Physiology and Behavior, 2*(119), 9-16.

10 Geliebter, A., Astbury, N. M., Aviram-Friedman, R., Yahav, E., & Hashim, S. (2014). Skipping breakfast leads to weight loss but also elevated cholesterol compared with consuming daily breakfasts of oat porridge or frosted cornflakes in overweight individuals: a randomised controlled trial. *Journal of Nutritional Sciences, 13*(3), 56.

11. Wishnofsky, M. (1958). Caloric equivalents of gained or lost weight. *American Journal of Clinical Nutrition, 6*(5), 542-6.

12. Tinsley, G. M., Forsse, J. S., Butler, N. K., Paoli, A., Bane, A. A., La Bounty, P. M., ... Grandjean, P. W. (2017). Time-restricted feeding in young men performing resistance training: A randomized controlled trial. *European Journal of Sport Science, 17*(2), 200-7.

13. Trabelsi, K., Stannard, S. R., Ghlissi, Z., Maughan, R. J., Kallel, C., Jamoussi, K., ... Hakim, A. (2013). Effect of fed – versus fasted state resistance training during Ramadan on body composition and selected metabolic parameters in bodybuilders. *Journal of the International Society of Sports Nutrition, 10*(1), 23-85.

14. Chakravarthy, M. V., Booth, F. W. (2004). Eating, exercise, and "thrifty" genotypes: Connecting the dots toward an evolutionary understanding of modern chronic diseases. *Journal of Applied Physiology, 96*(1), 3-10.

15. Mattson, M. P., & Wan, R. (2005). Beneficial effects of intermittent fasting and caloric restriction on the cardiovascular and cerebrovascular systems. *The Journal of Nutritional Biochemistry, 16*(3), 129-37.

16. Aksungar, F. B., Topkaya, A. E., & Akyildiz, M. (2007). Interleukin-6, C-reactive protein and biochemical parameters during prolonged intermittent fasting. *Annals of Nutrition and Metabolism, 51*(1), 88-95.

17. Goodrick, C. L., Ingram, D. K., Reynolds, M. A., Freeman, J. R., & Cider, N. L. (1982). Effects of intermittent feeding upon growth and life span in rats. *Gerontology, 28,* 233-41.

18. Yamamoto, J., Kamata, S., Miura, A., Nagata, T., Kainuma, R., Ishii, I. (2015). Differential adaptive responses to 1 – or 2-day fasting in various mouse tissues revealed by quantitative PCR analysis. *FEBS Open Bio, 5,* 357-68.

19. Lee, J., Duan, W., Long, J. M., Ingram, D. K., & Mattson, M. P. (2000). Dietary restriction increases the number of newly generated neural

cells, and induces BDNF expression, in the dentate gyrus of rats. *Journal of Molecular Neuroscience, 15*(2), 99-108.

20. Mattson, M. P. (2005). Energy intake, meal frequency, and health: A neurobiological perspective. *Annual Review of Nutrition, 25,* 237-60.

21. Varady, K. A., Bhutani, S., Church, E. C., & Kiempel, M. C. (2009). Short-term modified alternate-day fasting: A novel dietary strategy for weight loss and cardioprotection in obese adults. *American Journal of Clinical Nutrition, 90*(5), 1138-43.

22. Chaix, A., Zarrinpar, A., Miu, P., Panda, S. (2014). Time-restricted feeding is a preventative and therapeutic intervention against diverse nutritional challenges. *Cell Metabolism, 20*(6), 991-1005.

23. Furmli, S., Elmasry, R., Ramos, M., Fung, J. (2018). Therapeutic use of intermittent fasting for people with type 2 diabetes as an alternative to insulin. *BMJ Case Reports.* doi:10.1136/bcr-2017-221854

24. Brandhorst, S., Longo, V. D. (2016). Fasting and caloric restriction in cancer prevention and treatment. *Metabolism in Cancer, 207,* 241-66.

25. Mattson, M. P., Wan, R. (2005). Beneficial effects of intermittent fasting and caloric restriction on the cardiovascular and cerebrovascular systems. *The Journal of Nutritional Biochemistry, 16*(3), 129-37.

26. Heilbronn, L. K., Civitarese, A. E., Bogacka, I., Smith, S. R., Hulver, M., Ravussin, E. (2005). Glucose tolerance and skeletal muscle gene expression in response to alternate day fasting. *Obesity Research, 13*(3), 574-81.

27. Martin, B., Pearson, M., Kebejian, L. M., Golden, E., Keselman, A., Bender, M.,…Mattson, M. P. (2007). Sex-dependent metabolic, neuroendocrine, and cognitive responses to dietary energy restriction and excess. *Endocrinology, 148*(9), 4318-33.

28. Martin, B., Pearson, M., Brenneman, R., Golden, E., Wood, W., Prabhu, V.,…Maudsley, S. (2009). Gonadal transcriptome alterations in response to dietary energy intake: Sensing the reproductive environment. *PLoS One, 4*(1), E4146.

29. Petre, A. (2019, October 1). Does Calorie Counting Work? A Critical Look. Retrieved from https://www.healthline.com/nutrition/does-calorie-counting-work.

30. Hartmann-Boyce, J., Johns, D. J., Jebb, S. A., Aveyard, P. (2014). Effect of behavioural techniques and delivery mode on effectiveness of weight management: Systematic review, meta-analysis and meta-regression. *Obesity Reviews, 15*(7), 598-609.

31. Weigle, D. S., Breen, P. A., Matthys, C. C., Callahan, H. S., Meeuws, K. E., Burden, V. R., Purnell, J. Q. (2005). A high-protein diet induces sustained reductions in appetite, ad libitum caloric intake, and body weight despite compensatory changes in diurnal plasma leptin and ghrelin concentrations. *American Journal of Clinical Nutrition, 82*(1), 41-8.

32. Frary, J. M., Bjerre, K. P., Glintborg, D., Ravn, P. (2016). The effect of dietary carbohydrates in women with polycystic ovary syndrome: A systematic review. *Minerva Endocrinology, 41*(1), 57-69.

33. Juanola-Falgarona, M., Salvado, J., Jurado, N., Soler, A., Lopez, A., Ferré, M., ... Bullo, M. (2014). Effect of the glycemic index of the diet on weight loss, modulation of satiety, inflammation, and other metabolic risk factors: A randomized controlled trial. *American Journal of Clinical Nutrition, 100*(1), 27-35.

34. Goss, A. M., Chandler-Laney, P. C., Ovalle, F., Goree, L. L., Azziz, R., Desmond, R. A., ... Gower, B. A. (2014). Effects of a eucaloric reduced-carbohydrate diet on body composition and fat distribution in women with PCOS. *Metabolism, 63*(10), 1257-64.

35. Witbracht, M., Keim, N. L., Forester, S., Widaman, A., Laugero, K. (2015). Female breakfast skippers display a disrupted cortisol rhythm and elevated blood pressure. *Physiology & Behavior, 2015*(140), 215-21.

36. Scheer, F. A., Morris, C. J., & Shea, S. A. (2013). The Internal Circadian Clock Increases Hunger and Appetite in the Evening Independent of Food Intake and Other Behaviors. Obesity, 21(3), 421-423.

37. Farshchi, H. R., Taylor, M. A., Macdonald, I. A. (2004). Regular meal frequency creates more appropriate insulin sensitivity and lipid profiles compared with irregular meal frequency in healthy lean women. *European Journal of Clinical Nutrition, 58*(7), 1071-7.

38. Witbracht, M., Keim, N. L., Forester, S., Widaman, A., Laugero, K. (2015). Female breakfast skippers display a disrupted cortisol rhythm and elevated blood pressure. *Physiology & Behavior, 140*(7), 215-21.

39. Masihy, M., Monrroy, H., Borghi, G., Pribic, T., Galan, C., Nieto, A., ... Azpiroz, F. (2019). Influence of Eating Schedule on the Postprandial Response: Gender Differences. *Nutrients, 11*(2), 40-10.

40. Farshchi, H. R., Taylor, M. A., Macdonald, I. A. (2004). Decreased thermic effect of food after an irregular compared with a regular

meal pattern in healthy lean women. *International Journal of Obesity Related Metabolic Disorders, 28*(5), 653-60.

41. Farshchi, H. R., Taylor, M. A., Macdonald, I. A. (2004). Regular meal frequency creates more appropriate insulin sensitivity and lipid profiles compared with irregular meal frequency in healthy lean women. *European Journal of Clinical Nutrition, 58*(7), 1071-7.

42. Ribeiro, M., Lopez de Figueroa, P., Blanco, F. J., Mendes, A. F., Carames, B. (2016). Insulin decreases autophagy and leads to cartilage degradation. *Osteoarthritis Cartilage, 24*(4), 731-9.

43. Soeters, M. R., Lammers, N. M., Dubbelhuis, P. F., Ackermans, M., Jonkers-Schuitema, C. F., Fliers, E., ... Serlie, M. J. (2009). Intermittent fasting does not affect whole-body glucose, lipid, or protein metabolism. *The American Journal of Clinical Nutrition, 90*(5), 1244-1251.

44. Stern, S. B., Bleicher, S. J., Flores, A., Gombos, G., Recitas, D., Shu, J. (1976). Administration of aspartame in non-insulin-dependent diabetics. *Journal of Toxicology an Environmental Health, 2*(2), 429-439.

45. Anton, S. D., Martin, C. K., Han, H., Coulon, S., Cefalu, W. T., Geiselman, P., Williamson, D. A. (2010). Effects of stevia, aspartame, and sucrose on food intake, satiety, and postprandial glucose and insulin levels. *Appetite, 55*(1), 37-43.

46. Evert, A. B., Boucher, J. L., Bouche, Cypress, M., Dunbar, S. A., Franz, M. J., Mayer-Davis, E. J., ... Yancy, W. S. (2013). Nutrition Therapy Recommendations for the Management of Adults with Diabetes. *Diabetes Care, 36*(11), 3821-3842.

47. Magnuson, B. A., Burdock, G. A., Doull, J., Kroes, R. M., Marsh, G. M., Pariza, M. W., ... Williams, G. M. (2007). Aspartame: A safety evaluation based on current use levels, regulations, and toxicological and epidemiological studies. *Critical Reviews in Toxicology, 37*(8), 629-727.

48. Tandel, K. R. (2011). Sugar substitutes: Health controversy over perceived benefits. *Journal of Pharmacology & Pharmacotherapeutics, 2*(4), 236-243.

49. Heilbronn, L. K. (2005). Alternate-day fasting in nonobese subjects: Effects on body weight, body composition, and energy metabolism. *American Journal of Clinical Nutrition, 81*(1), 69-73.

50. Tiwari, S., Riazi, S. M., Ecelbarger, C. A. (2007). Insulin's impact on renal sodium transport and blood pressure in health, obesity, and diabetes. *American Journal of Physiology-Renal Physiology, 293*(4), F974-84.

51. EFSA Panel on Dietetic Products, Nutrition, and Allergies (NDA). (2010). Scientific Opinion on Dietary Reference Values for water. *EFSA Journal, 8(*3), 1459.
52. Vieux, F., Maillot, M., Constant, F., Drewnowski, A. (2016). Water and beverage consumption among children aged 4-13 years in France: Analyses of INCA 2 (Étude Individuelle Nationale des Consommations Alimentaires 2006-2007) data. *Public Health Nutrition, 19*(13), 2305-14.

Printed in Great Britain
by Amazon